JUICING FOR DIABETICS:

Best Recipes & Tips

Janet martins

Contents

DISCLAIMER:

All content is provided as general information only, and should not be taken as medical advice or professional guidance. Please consult with a qualified healthcare provider if you have any questions or concerns about your individual situation.

INTRODUCTION

Living with diabetes doesn't mean you have to give up your favorite foods. In fact, juicing for people with diabetes can be a great way to get all the nutrients you need while still enjoying your favorite flavors. In this book, we will discuss some of the best recipes for juicing for diabetics, as well as some tips on making the most of your juices. So whether you are just starting on your journey to better health or you are a seasoned juicer, we have something for everyone!

If you have diabetes, you know regulating your blood sugar levels is important. One way to do this is by eating healthy foods and drinks. Juicing can be a great way to get the nutrients your body needs and help regulate blood sugar levels.

If you are looking for ways to support your diabetes with juicing, you have come to the right place! This book will share some of the best recipes and tips to help get you started. Juicing can be a great way to get more nutrients into your diet and help regulate blood sugar levels. With these delicious recipes and helpful tips, you'll be on your way to better health in no time!

WHAT IS JUICING?

Juicing is extracting juice from plant tissues such as fruit or vegetables. Today, juicing is the given name to a new nutrition method, in which you consume mostly vegetable juices. Sometimes it's also called green juicing since it contains lots of green vegetables and has the color green. But there are better ways to name it than this because juicing is very colorful if you look at the original content.

Is Juicing Useful or a Temporary Trend?

Pilates, Zumba, and Soul Cycle studios have sprung up on every corner in recent years, and almost every gym has upgraded to accommodate these activities. Following this fad in physical fitness, a similar one has emerged in the food industry. Raw food restaurants, juicing businesses, organic grocery stores, and eateries serving alkaline waters are all rising.

Rather than labeling something as fleeting or a fad, we may describe it as the first step toward transformation after enlightenment. We realized that a healthy lifestyle requires a good diet, regular exercise, a sound body, and a tranquil state of mind. The progression from "Horse, lady, a weapon" to "Mind, body, soul" is rather dramatic. What's in our food is increasingly a pressing concern. For ethical and health reasons, we refuse to consume industrially produced foods. We'd rather not have to treat brand-new illnesses or newly developed sensitivities with medicine. Our goal is to eliminate them. We want to stop letting other people dictate how our bodies function.

To say this is just a fad would be to deny the awakening, and it would prove we haven't learned anything. So put, people can't give up the healthy ethos. Humans have a natural urge to save their own lives by taking measures to prevent harm to their health. Nonetheless, juicing's present popularity is rather recent. As juicing becomes commonplace, it will lose its novelty and become another meal.

Drinking or Eating?

To begin, in contrast to eating, drinking provides several benefits, including the following. You will only get hungry if all you do is drink full pineapple juice every day, but trying to eat every day can turn into a living nightmare for you. Consuming juice on a regular basis by drinking is unquestionably a lot more convenient than eating it. If you consume fruits and vegetables, the indigestible fiber will slow the absorption process to roughly 17 percent over three to five hours. But, the absorption is accelerated by up to 68% when you drink it, and the process takes just around 10 to 15 minutes.

In many ways, drinking juice is like taking a nutritional supplement. Within twenty minutes, the body will begin to process any food consumed. Juicing has an absorption rate of around 99%, but eating only halves the nutrients that even a person can absorb with the most efficient digestive system. In addition, the energy normally spent on digestion is not required while drinking juice, unlike when you are eating solid food.

It is common knowledge that heating tomatoes result in a fivefold increase in the antioxidant power of lycopene. Still, it is also common knowledge that was blending tomatoes results in the same effect.

In addition to the vitamins, enzymes, and minerals they supply, the primary benefit of eating fruits and vegetables is providing something of critical significance. It is impossible to sustain life without water. It is common knowledge that people can withstand hunger but not thirst. Water makes up around 65 percent of a person's total body mass. There are organs in which this rate is even much greater than this. As an example, the rate of this activity is 80% in the brain. Even though the significance of water in our lives is readily obvious, a significant number of us still do not drink enough of it. On the contrary, individuals drink less water these days because they are substituting other liquid beverages for water, such as tea, coffee, soda, and cola. This is causing their bodies to have less water overall.

In addition to their high water content, the vitamins, and minerals included in fruit and vegetable juices are among the most significant aspects of this beverage type. For example, although carrot juice supplies us with vitamin A in beta carotene, citrus fruits like grapefruit, oranges, and lemons are natural sources of vitamin C. Carrot juice also provides us with beta carotene. In addition, most green juices are fortified with vitamin E. Fruit and vegetable juices provide iron, copper, potassium, sodium, iodine, magnesium, and other essential minerals. In addition, the minerals obtained through juicing are more easily assimilated by the body during the digestion process when compared to the minerals obtained through eating.

When we juice, we absorb more nutrients than when we consume the same amount of food because the indigestible fibers are removed throughout the juicing process. To illustrate this point, if we eat a carrot, we only absorb 1% of the beta-carotene it contains due to indigestible fibers. On the other hand, if we drink raw carrot juice, we can absorb practically all of its beta-carotene.

The enzymes may also be obtained significantly from freshly extracted fruit and vegetable juices since they are damaged when heat exposure, and fruits and vegetables must be consumed when fresh. At temperatures higher than 114 degrees Fahrenheit, the cooking process kills the enzymes in food. However, since there will be no heat throughout the juicing process, all the enzymes will be active.

Raw food and juicing are still employed in various therapeutic practices in the modern period. There is a clear indication of progress being made in this area.

BENEFITS OF JUICING

Enhances your immune system is your body's natural defense against infection and disease. The stronger the system, the better equipped it is to fight unwanted invaders.

1. Delivers minerals and vitamins to the bloodstream

A healthy diet is important for many reasons, but did you know that what you eat can also affect the health of your blood? That's right, the nutrients in your food nourish your body and play a vital role in keeping your blood flowing smoothly. One way to make sure your blood gets the nutrients it needs is by juicing.

Juicing delivers minerals and vitamins directly to the bloodstream, which helps to keep the blood flowing properly. Minerals such as iron and copper are essential for producing red blood cells, while vitamins like vitamin C help to keep the blood vessels healthy. In addition, juicing can help to improve circulation by increasing the amount of oxygen in the blood.

1. Neutralizes bodies pH

A daily juicing habit can profoundly impact your health by helping to neutralize your body's pH. While the body is designed to maintain a slightly alkaline pH, modern diet and lifestyle choices tend to promote acidity. This can lead to serious health problems over time. But by including plenty of alkalizing fruits and vegetables in your juicing recipes, you can help offset the acidic foods and drinks you consume. This can help protect your bones and teeth, improve digestion, reduce inflammation, and boost your energy levels. So if you're looking for a simple way to improve your health, start incorporating more fresh juice into your diet!

Help reduce high levels of bad cholesterol and high blood pressure.

Juicing can help reduce high levels of bad cholesterol and high blood pressure, two factors leading to serious health problems.

Adding fresh fruits and vegetables to your diet is always a good idea, but juicing them can help ensure you get all the nutrients they contain. When you juice fruits and vegetables, your body can absorb their vitamins, minerals, and antioxidants more easily. These nutrients can help keep your heart healthy and lower your risk of developing cardiovascular disease. Not only will you be getting more of the healthy nutrients your body needs, but you may also be able to lower your cholesterol and blood pressure levels.

1. Combat eating disorders

Eating disorders and other problems are linked to physical and mental health issues. Overcoming such disorders as binge eating has become a serious issue. To stop binge eating, you need a regular eating pattern. So, including juices in your diet works well to stop binge eating. Including fruit juices like grapefruit juice can help overcome binge eating.

1. Improves energy levels

Many people are looking for a way to improve their energy levels. Whether working long hours, caring for a family, or attending school, we all need help getting through the day. That's where juicing comes in.

Not only does juicing give you the nutrients your body needs to function properly, but it can also help improve your energy levels. This is because when you juice, your body doesn't have to work hard to break the fruits and vegetables into usable nutrients.

So if you're looking for a natural way to boost your energy levels, try juicing! You'll be surprised at how much difference it can make.

1. Easy way to add fruits and vegetables to your diet

Daily juicing has many benefits, including high amounts of fruits and vegetables. Juicing allows you to consume more fruits and vegetables than you typically would eat in a day. This increase in consumption has many benefits for your health, including improved digestion, increased metabolism, and greater nutrient absorption.

In addition to the health benefits of juicing, you'll also enjoy the great taste of fresh juice. Juicing allows you to experiment with different flavor combinations to find the ones you love. With so many delicious and nutritious options, there's no reason not to start juicing today!

1. Hydrates your body

Your body is mostly made up of water; therefore, staying hydrated is crucial for optimal health. When you juice, you're getting the water from the fruits and vegetables and the nutrients and vitamins essential for proper hydration.

Juicing is an excellent way to help your body stay hydrated, especially if you struggle to drink enough water throughout the day. Not only does juicing provide your body with the fluids it needs, but it also helps to flush out toxins and promote healthy digestion.

1. Slows and, in some cases, even reverses the signs of aging.

Drinking freshly juiced fruits and vegetables has countless health benefits, including slowing and, in some cases, even reversing the signs of aging. Here's how it works:

The body absorbs the nutrients in fresh juice, so it can go to work immediately, repairing damage and boosting cell turnover. This helps to keep skin looking young and radiant.

Fresh juice is also packed with antioxidants, which help protect cells from damage caused by free radicals. Free radicals are one of the main culprits behind premature aging, so getting plenty of antioxidants is crucial for maintaining a youthful appearance. Plus, the vitamins add glow to your skin.

1. Detoxifies the body

Drinking freshly juiced fruits and vegetables is one of the best things you can do for your body. Not only does it provide you with vitamins, minerals, and antioxidants, but it also helps to cleanse and detoxify your system.

One of the main benefits of juicing is that it helps to flush out toxins from your body. This is because the juice's nutrients help stimulate your liver and promote healthy digestion. Additionally, juicing can help to improve your skin health by helping to eliminate toxins through your pores.

1. Help reduce weight

Obesity is an epidemic that has led to increased chronic diseases such as type 2 diabetes, heart disease, and stroke. People are finding new ways to lose weight, and one of the best ways is y adding natural ingredients to your diet. One way to help reduce weight is by juicing. Juicing can help people lose weight by providing a calorie-controlled diet and nutrients that promote satiety and help with weight loss. For example, one study found that participants who drank freshly squeezed vegetable juices daily lost more weight than those who didn't juice at all.

Juicing provides many benefits, including improved digestion, energy, detoxification, and clearer skin. Juicing is a great way to get your body's nutrients in a delicious and easy-to-consume form. If you are looking for a way to improve your health, juicing is a great option.

WHAT IS DIABETES

Diabetes is a disorder that develops when a person has an abnormally high level of sugar (glucose) in their blood. The condition manifests itself either when the pancreas fails to produce enough insulin or any insulin at all or when the body fails to react appropriately to the effects of insulin. Diabetes is a condition that may strike anyone at any age. Most diabetes types are chronic, which means they last a person's whole life. However, all kinds of diabetes may be managed with medicine and adjustments in lifestyle.

Sugar, or glucose, is mostly derived from the carbs in the diet. It is the primary source of fuel that your body uses. All of the cells in your body have access to glucose, which may be used as a source of energy.

When glucose is present in your bloodstream, it must assist with a key for key to reaching its ultimate destination. Insulin is the secret here (a hormone). If your pancreas isn't producing enough insulin or your body isn't utilizing it correctly, glucose will accumulate in your bloodstream, which will cause your blood sugar level to be too high (hyperglycemia).

Maintaining a blood glucose level that is continually high may eventually lead to a variety of health complications, including coronary heart disease, nerve damage, and vision impairments.

Diabetes mellitus is the medical term that's used to refer to diabetes. Diabetes insipidus is a condition that bears the name "diabetes," although the two conditions are not the same. Both conditions, which induce increased thirst and a need to urinate more often, are called diabetes. Diabetes insipidus is a condition that is diagnosed significantly less often than diabetes mellitus.

WHAT ARE THE TYPES OF DIABETES?

There are several types of diabetes. The most common forms include:

- Type 2 diabetes: With this type, your body doesn't make enough insulin, and your body's cells don't normally respond to the insulin (insulin resistance). This is the most common type of diabetes. It mainly affects adults, but children can have it as well.

- Prediabetes: This type is the stage before Type 2 diabetes. Your blood glucose levels are higher than normal but not high enough to be officially diagnosed with Type 2 diabetes.

- Type 1 diabetes is an autoimmune disease in which your immune system attacks and destroys insulin-producing cells in your pancreas for unknown reasons. Up to 10% of people who have diabetes have Type 1. It's usually diagnosed in children and young adults but can develop at any age.
- Gestational diabetes: This type develops in some people during pregnancy. Gestational diabetes usually goes away after pregnancy. However, if you have gestational diabetes, you're at a higher risk of developing Type 2 diabetes later in life.

Other types of diabetes include:

- Type 3c diabetes: This form of diabetes happens when your pancreas experiences damage (other than autoimmune damage), which affects its ability to produce insulin.

Pancreatitis, pancreatic cancer, cystic fibrosis, and hemochromatosis can all lead to pancreas damage that causes diabetes. Having your pancreas removed (pancreatectomy) also results in Type 3c.

- Latent autoimmune diabetes in adults (LADA): Like Type 1 diabetes, LADA also results from an autoimmune reaction but develops much more slowly than Type 1. People diagnosed with LADA are usually over the age of 30.

- Maturity-onset diabetes of the young (MODY): MODY, also called monogenic diabetes, happens due to an inherited genetic mutation that affects how your body makes and uses insulin. There are currently over 10 different types of MODY. It affects up to 5% of people with diabetes and commonly runs in families.

- Neonatal diabetes is a rare form of diabetes that occurs within the first six months of life. It's also a form of monogenic diabetes. About 50% of babies with neonatal diabetes have the lifelong form called permanent neonatal diabetes mellitus. The condition disappears within a few months from the onset for the other half but can come back later in life. This is called transient neonatal diabetes mellitus.

- Brittle diabetes: Brittle diabetes is a form of Type 1 diabetes marked by frequent and severe episodes of high and low blood sugar levels. This instability often leads to hospitalization. In rare cases, a pancreas transplant may be necessary to treat brittle diabetes permanently.

WHAT CAUSES DIABETES?

Too much glucose circulating in your bloodstream causes diabetes, regardless of the type. However, the reason why your blood glucose levels are high differs depending on the type of diabetes.

Causes of diabetes include:

- **I**nsulin resistance: Type 2 diabetes mainly results from insulin resistance. Insulin resistance happens when cells in your muscles, fat, and liver don't respond as they should to insulin. Several factors and conditions contribute to varying degrees of insulin resistance, including obesity, lack of physical activity, diet, hormonal imbalances, genetics, and certain medications.
- Autoimmune disease: Type 1 diabetes and LADA happen when your immune system

attacks the insulin-producing cells in your pancreas.

- Hormonal imbalances: During pregnancy, the placenta releases hormones that cause insulin resistance. You may develop gestational diabetes if your pancreas can't produce enough insulin to overcome insulin resistance. Other hormone-related conditions like acromegaly and Cushing syndrome can cause Type 2 diabetes.

- Pancreatic damage: Physical damage to your pancreas from a condition, surgery, or injury can impact its ability to make insulin, resulting in Type 3c diabetes.

- Genetic mutations: Certain genetic mutations can cause MODY and neonatal diabetes.

HOW IS DIABETES MANAGED?

Diabetes is a complex condition, so its management involves several strategies. In addition, diabetes affects everyone differently, so management plans are highly individualized.

The four main aspects of managing diabetes include:

- Blood sugar monitoring: Monitoring your blood sugar (glucose) is key to determining how well your current treatment plan works. It gives you information on how to manage your diabetes daily — and sometimes even hourly. You can regularly check your levels with a glucose meter, finger stick, and a continuous glucose monitor (CGM). You and your healthcare provider will determine your best blood sugar range.

- Oral diabetes medications: Oral diabetes medications (taken by mouth) help manage blood sugar levels in people with diabetes but still produce some insulin, mainly in people with Type 2 diabetes and prediabetes. People with gestational diabetes may also need oral medication. There are several different types. Metformin is the most common.

- Insulin: People with Type 1 diabetes must inject synthetic insulin to live and manage diabetes. Some people with Type 2 diabetes also require insulin. There are several different types of synthetic insulin. They each start to work at different speeds and last in your body for different lengths. The four main ways to take insulin include injectable insulin with a syringe (shot), insulin pens, insulin pumps, and rapid-acting inhaled insulin.

- Diet: Meal planning and choosing a healthy diet are key aspects of diabetes management, as food greatly impacts blood sugar. If you take insulin, counting carbs in your food and drinks is a large part of management. The amount of carbs you eat determines how much insulin you need at meals. Healthy eating habits can also help you manage your weight and reduce your heart disease risk.

- Exercise: Physical activity increases insulin sensitivity (and helps reduce insulin resistance), so regular exercise is an important part of management for all people with diabetes.

HOW CAN I PREVENT DIABETES?

You can't prevent autoimmune and genetic forms of diabetes. But there are some steps you can take to lower your risk for developing prediabetes, Type 2 diabetes, and gestational diabetes, including:

- Eat a healthy diet, such as the Mediterranean diet.
- Get physically active. Aim for 30 minutes a day, at least five days a week.
- Work to achieve a weight that's healthy for you.
- Manage your stress.
- Limit alcohol intake.
- Get adequate sleep (typically 7 to 9 hours) and seek treatment for sleep disorders.
- Quit smoking.
- Take medications as your healthcare provider directs to manage existing risk factors for heart disease.

THE BEST FOOD FOR DIABETES

1. Fatty fish

Fish, including salmon, sardines, herring, anchovies, and mackerel, are excellent providers of the omega-3 fatty acids DHA and EPA, all of which are associated with significant improvements in cardiovascular health when consumed regularly.

Those who have diabetes have a higher chance of developing cardiovascular disease and stroke. Thus they must consume an adequate amount of these fats daily.

The anti-inflammatory effects of DHA and EPA, together with the protection they provide to the cells that line your blood vessels, may improve your arteries' performance.

According to research, those who consume fatty fish daily have a decreased risk of acute coronary syndromes such as heart attacks and a reduced chance of passing away due to heart disease.

According to several studies, eating fish high in fat may also assist in maintaining normal blood sugar levels.

In a study that included 68 people who were overweight or obese, researchers discovered that those participants who ingested fatty fish had much better post-meal blood sugar levels than those who received lean fish.

Fish is an excellent source of high-quality protein, which makes you feel fuller for longer and contributes to maintaining stable blood sugar levels.

1. Leafy greens

Vegetables with a leafy green appearance have a low-calorie count and very high nutritional value.

They also include a relatively low amount of digestible carbohydrates, which are digested by the body, which means that they do not substantially alter blood sugar levels.

Vitamin C is one of the numerous vitamins and minerals that may be found in abundance in dark leafy greens like spinach, kale, and other similar greens.

Some evidence shows that persons with diabetes have lower levels of vitamin C than those who do not have diabetes, and they may have higher needs for vitamin C.

Vitamin C has powerful anti-inflammatory properties and its role as an antioxidant in the body.

Those who have diabetes may raise their blood vitamin C levels by increasing their dietary consumption of foods that are high in vitamin C. This can also help reduce inflammation and cellular damage.

1. **Avocados**

You don't need to worry about avocados raising your blood sugar levels since they contain less than 1 gram of sugar, very little carbs, a high fiber content, and healthy fats. Avocados also have a high fiber content.

Consumption of avocados has also been linked to an improvement in the quality of diet overall, as well as a considerable reduction in body weight and body mass index (BMI).

Because of this, people with diabetes should consider eating avocados as a snack, particularly considering the correlation between obesity and an increased risk of developing diabetes.

There is some evidence that eating avocados might help protect against diabetes.

In a research published in 2019, it was discovered that advocating B (AvoB), a lipid molecule that can only be found in avocados, decreases insulin resistance in skeletal muscle and the pancreas by inhibiting incomplete oxidation in both of those tissues.

1. Eggs

Consuming eggs regularly may lower the chance of developing heart disease in a number of different ways.

Eggs may reduce inflammation, enhance insulin sensitivity, raise HDL (good) cholesterol levels, and change the size and structure of LDL (bad) cholesterol. Eggs may also boost HDL (good) cholesterol levels.

According to the findings of research published in 2019, having a breakfast consisting mostly of eggs, which are rich in fat but low in carbohydrates may make it easier for persons with diabetes to control their blood sugar levels throughout the day.

An earlier study has associated egg intake with heart problems in patients with diabetes.

However, a more recent evaluation of controlled research indicated that eating 6 to 12 eggs per week as part of a balanced diet did not raise heart disease risk factors in adults with diabetes.

1. Chia seeds

Those who have diabetes may benefit greatly from eating chia seeds.

They have a very low digestible carbohydrate content and an extraordinarily high fiber content.

11 of the 12 grams of carbohydrates in a serving of chia seeds (equal to one ounce) are fiber, which does not cause an increase in blood sugar.

Chia seeds have a viscous fiber that may reduce your blood sugar levels. This happens because the viscous fiber slows down the pace at which food is absorbed and moved through the digestive tract.

Since fiber helps you feel full and suppresses your appetite, eating chia seeds can make it easier to maintain a healthy weight. In addition, Chia seeds have been shown to assist in maintaining proper glycemic regulation in diabetic patients.

Eating chia seeds was shown to assist weight reduction and help maintain excellent glycemic control in research that included 77 persons with type 2 diabetes who were overweight or obese and had been diagnosed with the condition.

1. **Beans**

Beans are affordable, nutritious, and super healthy.

Beans are a type of legume rich in B vitamins, beneficial minerals (calcium, potassium, and magnesium), and fiber.

They also have a very low glycemic index, which is important for managing diabetes.

Beans may also help prevent diabetes.

1. **Greek yogurt**

A daily serving of yogurt was associated with an 18 percent decreased risk of acquiring type 2 diabetes, according to large-scale, long-term research that included data on the participants' health from more than 100,000 people.

It may also assist you in achieving your specific objective of weight loss.

According to a number of studies, eating yogurt and other dairy products may help persons with type 2 diabetes lose weight and improve their overall body composition.

The high calcium and protein content in yogurt and the unique form of fat known as conjugated linoleic acid (CLA) can help you feel full for a longer period.

In addition, a serving of Greek yogurt only has between 6 and 8 grams of carbohydrates, much less than a serving of regular yogurt.

1. **Nuts**

Nuts are delicious and nutritious.

Most nuts contain fiber and are low in net carbs, although some have more.

Research on various nuts has shown that regular consumption may reduce inflammation and lower blood sugar, HbA1c (a marker for long-term blood sugar management), and LDL (bad) cholesterol levels.

Nuts may also help people with diabetes improve their heart health.

A 2019 study involving more than 16,000 participants with type 2 diabetes found that eating tree nuts such as walnuts, almonds, hazelnuts, and pistachios lowered their risk of heart disease and death.

1. Broccoli

Broccoli is one of the most nutritious vegetables around.

A half cup of cooked broccoli contains only 27 calories and 3 grams of digestible carbs and important nutrients like vitamin C and magnesium.

Broccoli may also help manage your blood sugar levels.

One study found that consuming broccoli sprouts led to a reduction in blood glucose in people with diabetes.

1. Extra-virgin olive oil

Extra-virgin olive oil contains oleic acid, a type of monounsaturated fat that may improve glycemic management, reduce fasting and post-meal triglyceride levels, and has antioxidant properties.

This is important because people with diabetes tend to have trouble managing blood sugar levels and have high triglyceride levels.

Oleic acid may also stimulate the fullness hormone GLP-1.

In a large analysis of 32 studies looking at different types of fat, olive oil was the only one shown to reduce heart disease risk.

Olive oil also contains antioxidants called polyphenols.

Polyphenols reduce inflammation, protect the cells lining your blood vessels, keep oxidation from damaging LDL (bad) cholesterol, and decrease blood pressure.

BEST JUICE RECIPES TO FIGHT DIABETES

The apple detox drink

This delicious **diabetic juice recipe** has a very healthy base that not only decreases the risk of diabetes and controls sugar but also has many other health benefits. The ingredients are:

- Two carrots
- One cup each of red apple and green apple, diced
- One lemon
- One one-inch block of ginger

Put all the ingredients through a juicer and serve fresh.

The Greenland drink

This is easily one of the **best juicing recipes for people with diabetes** since it has the goodness of all the major green veggies that are super detoxifiers and promote digestion. You can make this drink with:

- One bunch of chard
- Half a bunch of kale
- One small green cabbage
- One green apple
- Two celery ribs
- One lemon

Juice everything nicely and serve the drink fresh.

The veggie land drink

This is one of the super **juicing recipes for diabetics** that you will get hooked up to once you see the benefits to your body. The ingredients of this juice are as follows:

- One-and-a-half beet
- Four carrots
- Two tomatoes
- One clove of garlic

- One bunch of spinach

- Five romaine leaves

- Some parsley leaves

- Two celery ribs

- Some watercress

- Salt as per taste

Juice the ingredients well and mix salt at the end. The drink is ready to serve.

The bitter melon juice

This can be deemed a miracle fruit targeting high blood glucose levels. If you don't like its taste, you can add other fruits to the concoction. For the basic juice, you need:

- Two bitter melons

- Some water

You can either juice or blend them as per your preference and consume them fresh. Alternatively, you can juice the melons with cucumber, green apples, or lemons to make them taste better.

The sweet potato juice

This is another great option in the list of **diabetic juicing recipes** as it is full of fiber and good for maintaining the blood glucose content. You will need the following:

- One sweet potato
- One green apple
- Two celery ribs
- One one-inch block of ginger
- Some cinnamon powder

Juice all the ingredients and serve the drink fresh.

The broccoli juice

If you have type 2 diabetes, this is the perfect drink to supply Sulforaphane to the body for controlling glucose-producing enzymes. You will need the following:

- One broccoli head
- Two or more carrots as per the taste preference
- Two apples

Juice these ingredients and serve the drink fresh.

The tomato cleanser drink

All the goodness of tomatoes in the form of vitamins and minerals is abundant in this drink, and it significantly helps maintain heart health. You will need the following:

- Four big tomatoes, de-seeded
- A bunch of lettuce

Juice these two and serve the drink fresh.

The pepper magic drink

Antioxidants are very good at controlling sugar levels in the blood as they flush out toxins. This drink has plenty of antioxidants like lycopene. You need the following ingredients:

- One bunch of spinach leaves
- One red bell pepper or capsicum
- Two celery sticks
- One kiwi

Juice everything just fine, and the drink is ready.

The dandelion diabetic concoction

This is another gem among the great **diabetic juicing recipes** for type 2 diabetics that helps them with inflammation reduction and blood glucose reduction. This recipe includes the following ingredients:

- One big bunch of dandelion leaves
- Ten celery ribs
- Four green apples
- One lemon

Juice everything finely and serve the drink fresh.

The water magic

This is not an actual recipe, but the main idea is to consume a high amount of water to keep the body hydrated and detoxified. You can make the water intake even more exciting by adding certain fruits or herbs to it. It can be anything like-

- Lemon juice
- Cucumber juice or slices
- Fresh herbs
- Mint leaves
- Basil leaves
- Crushed berries

JUICING TIPS

THE BASICS

To begin, let's answer two points often asked: first, what is the difference between juice and a smoothie, and second, can juice be prepared using a blender?

During the juice extraction process, specialized machines separate the juice from the remaining solid matter, also known as the pulp, which is mostly composed of fiber. Juice that does not include pulp is more often recommended for weight reduction and general cleansing because of its pristine flavor and consistency. In contrast, a smoothie contains everything, including the juice and the peel of the fruit, and is thus a popular choice for cleansing the body and aiding digestion due to the increased fiber content of smoothies.

A blender with a lot of power is required to make a smoothie. Your regular blender at home will only be able to do the task if you are okay with a gritty mess that tastes more like an undercooked soup than a tasty beverage! On the other hand, if you have the time, you may use your blender and then strain the blended liquid through a coffee filter. This method is recommended only if you have the time. Smoothies and juices are equally delicious and wonderful for your health.

WHY JUICE?

People are becoming more interested in improving their health by drinking freshly squeezed juice. If you do a lot of traveling, you may have heard of a brand called "Joe & The Juice," which is gaining popularity in Europe at the same rate as Starbucks and is beginning to expand into the United States. And while we're on Starbucks, you've undoubtedly noticed that they've begun selling fresh juice.

Several scientific studies have shown that eating diets high in fruits and vegetables, such as the Mediterranean Diet, may lower the chance of getting a variety of ailments, including diabetes, cardiovascular disease, and even cancer. In addition, it is already common knowledge that certain types of fruits and vegetables may successfully cure various ailments, including Type 2 diabetes.

And that's not the end of it. Juicing can save you money. Since most of the same things can be found naturally in homemade juice, you no longer need to purchase those pricey multivitamins and other essential supplements.

Since juice that is sold commercially is required by law to be heated, a process known as pasteurization that impacts many nutrients, not even the greatest brand of bottled juice can come close to offering all the nutrients that may be found in the juice that is manufactured at home.

Store it, and you lose even more nutrients. In addition, many juices include sugar, colors, stabilizers, and other additions, all of which reduce the juice's potential nutritious value.

ARE THERE ANY DANGERS?

There are some issues if you're on medication, so be sure to speak with your doctor before juicing especially if you're on thyroid medications — certain foods interfere with your medication. And too much of the more powerful foods, such as greens or beets, can upset your stomach.

JUICE OR RAW?

Depending on the particular variety, there are benefits to drinking your daily recommended servings of veggies and fruits instead of eating them as solid raw foods. Liquids, in general, are absorbed by the body more quickly and completely. Solid food takes a slower path of absorption through the stomach and intestines, and you need to chew your food thoroughly to get as much nutrition from raw as you do from the liquid form in some cases.

Juice or Cooked

Cooking food may kill certain nutrients. For instance, enzymes play a key role in metabolism and are chiefly found in raw foods, but most are lost when cooked, processed, and preserved. Enzymes are particularly important for digestion.10 Interestingly, some nutrients are enhanced by steaming, such as lycopene in tomatoes.

JUICE BENEFITS

Increased energy and possible weight loss are not the only benefits of fresh juice. Recent research suggests that drinking fresh juice, like oranges, can also delay the effects of aging. Specifically, fresh fruits and vegetables contain compounds known as antioxidants which neutralize free radicals in your body. Free radicals are chiefly responsible for aging and many degenerative diseases such as cataracts, high blood pressure, and even cancer.

Fight Disease

Let's explore how juicing affects one of our most common chronic diseases: diabetes. Research indicates that certain raw fruits and vegetables nourish the body while stabilizing blood sugar levels, largely due to the insoluble fiber in whole vegetables. While juices with added sugar should be avoided, 100% fruit juice was not associated with the risk of developing type 2 diabetes.

Additional research also found that specific nutrients such as vitamins A, B, E, and the minerals iron and potassium, which are abundant in fresh fruits and vegetables, aid in naturally managing this disease. Vitamin B7, which is found in mangoes, nectarines, and peaches, aids in digestion and activates enzymes, which are particularly helpful for people with diabetes. Additionally, manganese found in celery, garlic, carrots, cruciferous vegetables, parsley, spinach, and beet greens helps reduce insulin resistance overall and improve sugar metabolism.

Juice Machines

What's the best machine? You can easily begin with an inexpensive juicer sold online or at your local kitchen supply store. We highly recommend the newer generation of machines known as 'slow' juicers because they reduce the amount of heat and oxygen in your juice factors that affect nutrients. They are also easier to clean and durable.

IS DRINKING JUICE A GOOD IDEA FOR PEOPLE WITH TYPE 2 DIABETES?

Those who do not have type 2 diabetes often do not give drinking a glass of juice a second thought when given the opportunity. But, on the other hand, this may not be the wisest choice for those who have type 2 diabetes.

When a person develops diabetes, it interferes with their body's ability to convert the fuel from their food into usable energy. For instance, once you eat anything, that meal will eventually be broken down into sugar and released into the blood. This process occurs regardless of what you eat. When there is a rise in this blood sugar, a signal is sent to the pancreas to produce insulin. Insulin can assist blood sugar in entering cells to be utilized for energy.

On the other hand, if you have diabetes, your body either does not produce enough insulin or cannot utilize the insulin it already has to draw blood sugar into cells so they can use it as a source of energy. Therefore, it is possible to end up with high blood sugar levels and other issues if the glucose levels in the blood are not brought down to a healthy range.

Fruits have a high fiber content, which makes them an excellent source of this beneficial vitamin since fiber slows down the pace at which the body absorbs glucose and sugar from the digestive system. But, when it comes to fruit juices, during the process of juicing, the majority of the fiber is removed, leaving primarily the sugar, which, when taken, may lead to a sudden and large jump in blood glucose levels. This is especially problematic for those who have diabetes.

While drinking juice won't create problems for most individuals, those with diabetes may not be able to consume this beverage owing to the possible hazards of the rapid blood sugar levels that diabetes patients experience.

WHAT ARE THE BENEFITS AND DRAWBACKS OF DRINKING JUICE FOR TYPE 2 DIABETES?

Many people like beginning their mornings with a glass of juice, and it's easy to see why. Nonetheless, moderation in juice consumption is always recommended regardless of whether or not a person has diabetes. This is because fruit juices often have many calories per serving, include more sugar than what is considered healthy for daily intake, and lack the fiber in whole fruits.

Why do individuals still go for a glass of juice when they want to nibble on something that's good for them? This is often the case because, depending on the kind of fruit juice, it may bring various advantages. Even those who have type 2 diabetes may be able to take advantage of some of these benefits.

For instance, fruit juice is a fantastic source of vitamin C, a nutrient required for growth, as well as the maintenance and repair of bodily tissues. In addition to these benefits, it aids in the formation of collagen, iron absorption, and the immune system's healthy operation.

According to a number of studies, eating vegetables and drinking fruit juices may be associated with a reduced risk of developing a number of different types of chronic illnesses, including cardiovascular diseases, malignancies, and neurological disorders. The findings of this study indicate that the cardiovascular system, including the heart, may benefit from consuming juices made from fruits and vegetables.

Several people also decide to get these advantages by consuming juices for this reason. In addition, the daily guidelines for vitamins, minerals, and antioxidants may substantially impact a person's health. Therefore, this method is often a quicker and more condensed approach to fulfill those requirements.

For instance, fruit juice made entirely from fruit includes bioactive chemicals with antioxidant activity, which may increase both the antioxidant status and the blood lipid levels.

However, even though a person can meet their daily vitamin C requirement by drinking a cup of orange juice, eating fruits and vegetables should still be the preferred method of reaching the desired intake of this nutrient. This is especially true when considering all the negative aspects of drinking juice. Those with type 2 diabetes who eat excessive juice drinks, for instance, may struggle with both weight gain and hyperglycemia due to their drinking habits.

Hyperglycemia, which occurs when there is a sudden rise in the amount of sugar in the blood, is linked to a number of potentially life-threatening disorders, including the following:

1) hyperosmolar hyperglycemic state leading to severe bodily dehydration, and

2) diabetic ketosis, which can lead to coma.

Chronic hyperglycemia can damage certain body parts, including the eyes, kidneys, nerves, and blood vessels. Damage to these blood vessels can also increase your risk of a stroke or a heart attack and delay wound healing.

If you are drinking juices, it is important to pay attention to hyperglycemia symptoms, including tiredness, blurred vision, increased thirst, dry mouth, and a general feeling of being unwell.

JUICE OPTIONS GOOD FOR TYPE 2 DIABETES

Even though people with type 2 diabetes are often advised to choose low-calorie drinks with low sugar, they can also drink juices. Take, for instance, the following:

Fruit juice

While it is generally advised to avoid fruit juices due to the high sugar content, it is best to consume juices with lower sugar content if needed.

This means opting for 100% natural juices with 0 added sugars and avoiding fruit juices made from pineapple or mangos. These fruit juices often have a significant amount of sugar. Instead, stick with unsweetened lemon or grapefruit juice, which has a lower glycemic index than most other juices.

Vegetable juice

Juices made from fresh vegetables are often better for type 2 diabetes because they usually have a lower glycemic index and a high amount of antioxidants.

Foods with a low glycemic index have been shown to control type 2 diabetes and aid with weight loss. As a result, for a healthy alternative, those with diabetes should try juices with kale and spinach, which are excellent at regulating blood sugar levels.

WHAT ARE THE BEST JUICES FOR TYPE 2 DIABETES?

If grapefruit juice is not your top drink choice, there are still other juices that may be a good option for those with type 2 diabetes, including:

Tomato juice

Tomato juice is a great choice for those who have type 2 diabetes. It has been known to reduce the risk of blood clots, a common issue for those with diabetes due to the associated risk of developing atherosclerosis and cardiovascular issues.

Pomegranate juice

This juice is rich in fiber, folate, and potassium and contains vitamin C. This juice is also loaded with specific types of antioxidants. Plus, because it has a low glycemic index, pomegranate juice is a good option for those with diabetes.

Studies[2] have reported that they are beneficial in controlling diabetes and some of its complications.

Carrot juice

Even though carrots have a sweet flavor, they can help manage blood glucose levels and, in moderation, won't spike blood sugar levels.

Carrots also contain minerals, vitamins, and carotenoids, which can serve as antioxidants and help the body. However, it's important to limit the portion of this juice as despite having a low glycemic index, a 250gm serving of carrot juice will contain 23gm of carbs.

BENEFITS OF JUICING FOR DIABETICS

1 . Provides essential vitamins and minerals: Juicing is a great way to get the essential vitamins and minerals you need for a healthy body, even for people with diabetes. The natural sugars in fruits and vegetables are slowly released into the bloodstream, making them a good choice for those with diabetes.

2. Manages blood sugar levels: People with diabetes must control their blood sugar levels within the normal range. Drinking freshly made juice that contains mostly fruits and vegetables can help stabilize your blood glucose levels and give you an energy boost if needed.

3. Reduces dependence on processed foods: Diabetics should avoid processed foods because they often contain added sugars or artificial sweeteners, which can harm health. Juicing helps to reduce dependence on processed foods and to increase the intake of fresh produce. This will help you ensure your diet is filled with essential nutrients needed for a healthy lifestyle.

4. Detoxifies the body: Juicing can help detoxify the body by flushing out toxins and helping break down fats accumulated due to unhealthy eating habits. This can be beneficial for people with diabetes, as it helps to regulate blood sugar levels and improve overall health.

5. Improves digestion: Drinking freshly made juices can also help improve digestion, which is important for people with diabetes who may experience digestive issues due to their condition.

The nutrients in juice can help aid digestion and promote regularity, improving overall health.

By adding freshly made juices to your diet, you can be sure that you are getting the necessary vitamins and minerals for a healthy lifestyle. Juicing for people with diabetes is a great way to get important nutrients while helping manage blood sugar levels. Considering these benefits, it's easy to see why juicing can benefit people with diabetes.

WHAT TO LOOK FOR WHEN CHOOSING FRUITS AND VEGETABLES

1 . Look for low-glycemic fruits and vegetables such as apples, oranges, grapefruits, pears, strawberries, blueberries, cranberries, broccoli, celery, and cucumbers.

2. Choose fruits and vegetables high in fiber, such as spinach, kale, and other dark leafy greens. Fiber slows down the digestion process, which helps to keep blood sugar levels balanced over time.

3. Avoid fruits with high sugar, such as bananas and mangoes.

4. Opt for seasonal produce when available to get the most nutrition from your juice combinations.

5. Avoid processed and packaged fruits, vegetables, and juices as they often contain added sugar and preservatives.

Following these guidelines, you can create delicious and nutritious juice combinations beneficial for managing diabetes without sacrificing taste or nutrition. Enjoy!

CONCLUSION

Juicing for people with diabetes is a great way to get essential vitamins and minerals and help manage blood sugar levels. It can reduce dependence on processed foods and help increase the intake of fresh produce, giving you the healthy nutrients needed to stay healthy. Juicing may also provide other benefits, such as improved digestion, increased energy levels, better skin health, and improved mental alertness, all while lowering your risk of complications from diabetes. With careful monitoring and smart decisions about what kinds of fruits and vegetables to juice, it can be an enjoyable part of managing diabetes. Start juicing today to take advantage of all the potential benefits.